RATION
CARE

RATION
CARE

JOHN AMAN

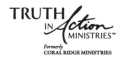

Fort Lauderdale, Florida

RationCare: The powerful unelected board that threatens health care in America

© 2012 Truth in Action Ministries

All rights reserved. Written permission must be secured from the publisher to use or reproduce any part of this book, except for brief quotations in critical reviews or articles.

All Scriptures are taken from the New King James Version. Copyright © 1982 by Thomas Nelson, Inc. Used by permission. All rights reserved.

Truth in Action Ministries
P.O. Box 1
Fort Lauderdale, FL 33302
1-800-988-7884
letters@tiam.org
www.TruthInAction.org

ISBN: 978-1-929626-08-3

CONTENTS

CHAPTER 1	Ruled by "Experts"	7
CHAPTER 2	RationCare Abroad	15
CHAPTER 3	RationCare At Home	23
CHAPTER 4	America's New "Rationing Board"	31
CHAPTER 5	Health Care in a Post-Christian World	41
ENDNOTES		49

CHAPTER 1

RULED BY "EXPERTS"

"The nine most terrifying words in the English language are, 'I'm from the government and I'm here to help.'"
—Ronald Reagan

People smile at former President Ronald Reagan's good-natured dig at those who believe government intervention is always the best option for any social crisis. There is something comic, albeit exasperating, about the naïve but well-intentioned liberal who believes he, and those like him, know best how to run America and bring an end to every social ill.

Yet things never work out quite as they were intended. President Lyndon B. Johnson earnestly announced the "War on Poverty" in 1964 with the confident declaration, "For the first time in our history, it is possible to conquer poverty." That turned out not to be the case. After spending some $17 trillion to win the war, the poor are still with us. One in seven Americans remains in poverty, according to the Census Bureau.[1]

Up until now, Americans have not had reason to be "terrified" by the ambitions of government elites. After all, big-spending social liberals seem to want good outcomes, even if their social improvement plans always go badly off track and fail to reach the intended objective.

But things have changed. Reagan's remark is not nearly so amusing now that Congress has passed the "Patient Protection and Affordable Care Act," a massive law that brings the health care industry—18 percent[2] of the American economy—under the close supervision of the federal government. Health policy expert Peter Ferrara calls it "nothing short of a government takeover of health care."[3]

NOT TOO STRONG A WORD

Suddenly "terrifying" is not too strong a word, when one contemplates the law's likely impact on the very ill, the elderly, and the unborn.[4] After all, the law brings sweeping changes to American health care, vests new powers in unelected bureaucrats, and is being implemented by elites who believe in the power of government while openly expressing support for health care rationing and the "freedom to choose" to kill unborn children.

It's bad enough that the law, rammed through Congress in 2010 against the will of the American people,[5] calls for $500 billion in new taxes over its first 10 years,[6] will cost $2.3 trillion in its first decade of full implementation,[7] will drive up the cost of premiums,[8] and will still leave some 23 million Americans uninsured.[9] It's even worse that the law cuts $575 billion from Medicare, which will leave seniors with fewer health care options as more doctors opt out of the underfunded system and decline Medicare patients.

Worst of all, the law gives an unelected board of 15 presidentially appointed and unaccountable "experts" the power to use price controls and other cuts to achieve spending reduction targets it prescribes. And there is very little Congress can do to stop the binding "recommendations" of this Independent Payment Advisory Board (IPAB) from taking effect.

Its proposals are law unless Congress says "No," which requires a majority House vote, an unlikely 60-vote Senate supermajority, and presidential approval.

Douglas Holtz-Eakin, a former director of the Congressional Budget Office, calls IPAB a "dramatic policy error that will fail to deliver meaningful reform to the Medicare program" and "possibly the most dangerous aspect of the Patient Protection and Affordable Care Act." He supports its immediate repeal,[10] as do 218 members of the U.S. House of Representatives who have co-sponsored H.R. 452, a measure to repeal IPAB.[11]

The threat from IPAB, Holtz-Eakin points out, is that in its effort to contain Medicare spending, "It will effectively determine that patients should have coverage for one particular treatment option, but not another, or must pay much more for one of the treatment options."[12]

NO APPEAL. NO REVIEW.

This central 15-member "payment board" will make decisions for millions of Medicare users about what procedures they may and may not have. And those decisions are final. If the board decides not to pay for a procedure you need, that decision is the last word. There is no appeal. Nor are IPAB's decisions subject to judicial review.

But that's not all. The law also empowers IPAB to advise Congress on how to reduce total private health care spending in America. Those recommendations are said to be non-binding, but an analysis from the National Right to Life Committee (NRLC) suggests otherwise, noting that the law gives the Secretary of Health and Human Services the power to effectively impose IPAB proposals on the private sector. According to the NRLC:

> This means that treatment that a doctor and patient deem advisable to save that patient's life or preserve or improve the patient's health, but which exceeds the standard imposed by the government, will be denied, even if the patient is willing and able to pay for it.[13]

Insulated from the reach of voters, and with a high legislative hurdle to any override of its edicts, IPAB almost guarantees, for the first time, a hard-cap on Medicare spending—something Congress has been unwilling to do. It is true that Medicare, as now structured, is unsustainable, but merely cutting payments will only worsen matters. Doing so means less care for seniors as doctors exit the Medicare system and IPAB makes decisions about what care Medicare will reimburse and what it will not.

Former Sens. John Breaux and Bill Frist warned, just before the health law's passage, that IPAB "would have the power to influence and rewrite nearly all aspects of Medicare."[14]

IPAB is the "real death panel"[15] in the new health care law says Rep. Phil Roe (R-TN), a physician who has practiced medicine for more than 30 years and has introduced legislation to repeal IPAB.

Rep. Pete Stark (D-CA) a congressional liberal who voted for the health care overhaul, called IPAB "a mindless rate-cutting machine that sets the program up for unsustainable cuts." On the same day that health care reform passed Congress, Stark warned that IPAB "will endanger the health of America's seniors and people with disabilities."[16]

Peter Orszag, who stepped down in 2011 as director of the Obama administration's Office of Management and Budget, is one of IPAB's biggest fans. He has called it a "very promising structure" for limiting Medicare costs and counts it a virtue that IPAB's decrees are very hard for Congress to overturn. Orszag is happy to take the hard questions in government away from politicians and let the "experts" call the shots:

> To solve the serious problems facing our country, we need to minimize the harm from legislative inertia by relying more on automatic policies and depoliticized commissions for certain policy decisions. In other words, radical as it sounds, we need to counter the gridlock of our political institutions by making them a bit less democratic.[17]

That's not exactly what the Founders had in mind when they

drafted our Constitution. For them, gridlock was a good thing. Since men are not angels, as James Madison said in "Federalist No. 51," reflecting a biblical worldview, the concentration of power in any one department of government must be resisted. "Ambition must be made to counteract ambition …," he wrote, in order to "… control the abuses of government."[18]

MADISON: DISTRUST THOSE IN POWER

Author Jerry Newcombe points out in his book, *Answers from the Founding Fathers*, that Madison, like the rest of the founding generation, was skeptical in the extreme of claims to human goodness and refused to rest power in the hands of a few. As Madison said, "All men having power ought to be distrusted."[19]

Thomas Jefferson shared that distrust. "The way to have good and safe government," said Jefferson, "is not to trust it all to one, but to divide it among the many…."[20]

Ben Franklin had the same view of humanity: "There is scarce a king in a hundred who would not, if he could, follow the example of Pharaoh, get first all the peoples' money, then all their lands and then make them and their children servants forever."[21]

The founders came to their settled conclusion about human sinfulness from Scripture, which declares:

> "There is none righteous, no, not one" (Romans 3:10);
>
> "For all have sinned and fall short of the glory of God" (Romans 3:23)
>
> "The heart is deceitful above all things, and desperately wicked; who can know it?" (Jeremiah 17:9).

The founders also understood the reality of human sinfulness due to what the Rev. John Witherspoon, Madison's instructor at Princeton and a signer of the Declaration of Independence, called "the inflexible testimony of daily experience…."[22]

It was because of the corruption of our nature, testified to by both the Scriptures and everyday life, that the founders established a system of divided government in the Constitution. They were wary of centralized power, as Madison explained in "Federalist No. 47":

> The accumulation of all powers, legislative, executive, and judiciary, in the same hands, whether of one, a few, or many, and whether hereditary, self-appointed, or elective, may justly be pronounced the very definition of tyranny.[23]

But Orszag wants less democracy in the form of "automatic policies and depoliticized commissions" and considers IPAB "perhaps the most dramatic example of this idea...." As he explains:

> The IPAB will be an independent panel of medical experts tasked with devising changes to Medicare's payment system. In each year that Medicare's per capita costs exceed a certain threshold, the IPAB is responsible for making proposals to reduce projected cost growth. The proposals take effect automatically unless Congress specifically passes legislation blocking them and the president signs that legislation.[24]

Orszag is not alone in his desire to remove sensitive choices from the political process.

Former Senate Majority Leader Tom Daschle, President Obama's first choice for Secretary of Health and Human Services, has praised the creation of IPAB because it makes possible the tough choices that Congress has dodged. "I can't think of anything in the ACA [Affordable Care Act] that is more important than ultimately giving some real authority to someone to make these tough decisions," Daschle said.[25]

Another former senator, Judd Gregg, a Republican from New Hampshire, agreed that there are some things Congress can not do. "There is no way, in a populist system that you can discuss the last six months of life," Gregg said at a health care reform debate with Daschle. "It's impossible. You do need some insulation from the political system to turn and address some of these complicated issues."[26]

Donald Berwick, the man President Obama named in a recess appointment to head the Centers for Medicare & Medicaid Services, the federal agency charged with implementing the new health care law, agrees with Orszag that it is up to the experts, not mere individual consumers, to resolve the complexities of modern health care.

Berwick, who has admitted he is "romantic" about Britain's National Health Service, believes health care rationing is inevitable and that wise and able leaders, not market forces, will bring us to what we "want and need" in health care.

"Do not trust market forces to give you the system you need...," said Berwick. "I cannot believe that the individual health care consumer can enforce through choice the proper configurations of a system as massive and complex as health care. That is for leaders to do."[27]

PERFECT EXPRESSION OF PROGRESSIVE MIND

Columnist George Will calls IPAB a "perfect expression of the progressive mind." IPAB illustrates, as does Berwick's comment above, what Will calls the essential doctrine of progressivism: "Modern society is too complex for popular sovereignty, so government of, by and for supposedly disinterested experts must not perish from the earth."[28]

But if "all men having power ought to be distrusted," as Madison said, we ought to intensely question whether the "experts" are in fact "disinterested." There may be other motives at work beyond the cheery claim that "I'm here to help."

Paul Starr, an advisor to Presidents Clinton and Obama, spoke of other ambitions that may be at work in his 1982 book, *The Social Transformation of American Medicine*:

> Political leaders since Bismarck seeking to strengthen the state or to advance their own or their party's interests have used insurance against the costs

of sickness as a means of turning benevolence to power.[29]

The late nineteenth century German Chancellor Otto von Bismarck presided over the birth of the modern welfare state, which included national health insurance, old-age pension, a minimum wage, workplace rules, vacation, and unemployment insurance, as a means to retain power. As Bismarck explained to an American visitor, "My idea was to bribe the working classes, or shall I say, to win them over, to regard the state as a social institution existing for their sake and interested in their welfare."[30]

Whatever their agenda, those who champion government as the best means to oversee or deliver health care—and introduce anti-democratic means like IPAB—must answer for the dismal record of such schemes elsewhere. The inevitable result of socialized medicine wherever it is tried is the "rationing of health care by people who will never even know our names."[31]

That's obvious from the troubling results of government-run health care systems in Britain and Canada. It's also evident in the health care rationing already taking place in Oregon and Massachusetts, two states where government has adopted an expanded role in the delivery of health care.

CHAPTER 2

RATIONCARE ABROAD

Britain has had socialized medicine since 1948. Its National Health Service is the world's largest government-run health provider and claims to be "one of the most efficient, most egalitarian and most comprehensive."[32]

That is open to serious doubt.

Wesley Smith, author of *Culture of Death: The Assault on Medical Ethics in America*, has visited England many times. In November 2011, he told Truth in Action Ministries, "If you look at what's happening in the NHS today with its constrained budgets—what do you see? You see women giving birth in hospital corridors. You see people waiting in ambulances for hours before they can get into an emergency room."[33]

In fact, nearly 4,000 women in Britain gave birth in places like hospital corridors, elevators, ambulances, even hospital toilets in 2008, due to a shortage of maternity beds.[34]

Faced with budget cuts, Britain's National Health Service now limits hip and knee replacement surgeries to patients in severe pain. Patients in need of cataract operations have to wait until their vision impairment "substantially" impacts their ability to work.[35]

Some six percent of Britons resort to self-dentistry, according to a 2007 survey of more than 5,000 people, some of whom reported using pliers to extract their own teeth.[36]

Self-dentistry is one thing. Surgery is another. Britons wait on the experts for that—and wait and wait. In May 2011, 2.54 million people were on a waiting list after being referred to a hospital for surgery.[37]

Despite NHS claims about its high-quality service, its ombudsman lashed out at the health system for "failing to meet even the most basic standards of care." He also gave the government-run health system low marks for an attitude, "both personal and institutional," which failed "to recognize the humanity and individuality of the people concerned and to respond to them with sensitivity, compassion and professionalism."[38]

DON'T CARE. DON'T HAVE TO.

That sounds like what they used to say about "Ma Bell," AT&T, which once enjoyed a government-sanctioned telephone monopoly: "We don't care. We don't have to."

Actual health care rationing decisions in the United Kingdom are made by a board called the National Institute for Health and Clinical Excellence (NICE). It determines whether a treatment may be offered by weighing the cost against the likely medical benefit. The most it will pay for one "Quality Adjusted Life Year" is about $45,000 and it has denied medicine to treat Alzheimer's and kidney patients.

NICE employs a sliding scale that rates the worth of one year of life higher for healthy people than for those who are sick. It also looks, author Sally Pipes explains,

> at how long a patient is likely to live with—and without—a given treatment, plus the success rate and cost of that treatment. If you happen to be a patient

in desperate need of a life-saving medicine, your fate depends on how NICE crunches the numbers.[39]

NICE denied treatments for leukemia patients in 2011. A press report said it ruled "three types of medication, which can give a normal life expectancy to patients with the rare blood cancer, are not effective enough, considering they cost up to £40,000 a year."[40]

Tom Daschle, who remained influential in the health care legislative battle, even after unpaid taxes scuttled his nomination to be HHS Secretary,[41] has long favored an American version of NICE. Dr. Scott Gottlieb wrote in a *Wall Street Journal* column in 2009 that Daschle

> argues that the only way to reduce spending is by allocating medical products based on "cost effectiveness." He's also called for a "federal health board" modeled on the Federal Reserve to rate medical products and create central controls on access.[42]

CANADIAN HEALTH CARE: GOING SOUTH

Canadians fare no better than Brits under socialized medicine. Canada's government-run system offers "free" universal health care to its citizens and is plagued by the same service and quality problems as Britain's NHS, which is why Newfoundland premier Danny Williams flew to Miami in February 2010 for heart surgery. Williams, a strong advocate of socialized medicine in Canada, told the Canadian Press that he crossed the border for surgery because "this was my heart, my choice and my health. I did not sign away my right to get the best possible health care for myself when I entered politics."[43]

Had he opted for treatment in Canada, it might have taken 18 weeks, the average wait time, after referral, for surgery in 2010.[44]

Thousands of Canadians have joined Williams in seeking health care in America. Shona Holmes was put on a waiting list to see a specialist for her failing eyesight. Rather than wait, the

Ontario resident traveled to a Mayo Clinic in Arizona, where she was quickly diagnosed with a brain tumor and received an operation in short order.

Had Holmes waited the two months or more it would have taken her to see a neurologist in Canada, she might have lost her sight. She had already lost half her sight in one eye and 25 percent of her vision in the other by the time she reached the Mayo Clinic, according to doctors there.[45]

Holmes told Truth in Action Ministries that, had she waited for treatment, "the absolute best case scenario that would've happened to me is I would've been permanently blind ... the worst case scenario is I wouldn't be sitting here today."[46]

And it's not just Canadian patients who are coming south. Canadian physicians are also doing so—not to seek treatment, but, rather, a better living—one reason for the doctor shortage also plaguing Canada. Author Sally Pipes cites data showing that Canada is now 26th in the number of doctors per thousand people on a list of 30 countries monitored by the Organization for Economic Cooperation and Development.[47] As a comparison, it ranked fourth in 1970, when the government became the nation's health care provider. Doctors in Canada earn 42 percent less, on average, than their counterparts in the U.S. Over the last ten years, some 10 percent of physicians trained in Canada have moved to the United States to earn more.[48]

But are the experiences of Britain and Canada relevant to our nation, now that the "Patient Protection and Affordable Care Act" has become law? After all, the new health care law does not entirely socialize medicine in America. We still have private insurance, private hospitals, and doctors in private practice. True, but it is a government "takeover," argues Peter Ferrara, a policy analyst and attorney who serves as general counsel for the America Civil Rights Union. Ferrara notes that the new law creates the infrastructure of more than 150 "bureaucracies, agencies, boards, commissions, and programs to rule over health care in America,"[49] among them the Independent Payment Advisory Board.

This "astonishing expansion" of government authority over

the heretofore mostly private American health sector includes, Ferrara notes, the power to

> tell doctors and hospitals what is quality health care and what is not, what are best practices in medicine, how their medical practices should be structured, and what they will be paid and when. Government authorities will mandate exactly what health insurance with what benefits workers and employers must buy, and the Act imposes tax penalties on them if they do not comply. Government authorities will dictate to insurance companies exactly what health insurance they must sell, to whom they must sell it, and what they can charge. Obamacare even redistributes premium income among insurers under a new "risk adjustment" mechanism. This adds up to nothing short of a government takeover of health care.[50]

Health care rationing will be the inevitable consequence of this government takeover. It's not necessary to look abroad for what happens when bureaucrats—not doctors—are in charge. Nor is it necessary to have an explicit system of "universal" health care.

WE'LL PAY YOU TO DIE

In 2008, after being diagnosed with prostate cancer, Randy Stroup asked Oregon's state-run health plan for chemotherapy treatment and got a letter back that "dropped my chin to the floor," as he told FOX News.

The state refused to cover his cancer treatment but did offer to pay for the cost of his physician-assisted suicide. Stroup's chances of survival were deemed too low, less than five percent, to justify the treatment, but under guidelines developed by Oregon's legislature, the pills and medical assistance needed to end Stroup's life could be covered.[51]

Another Oregonian, 64-year-old Barbara Wagner, got a similar answer when she asked the Oregon Health Plan to pay for

Tarceva, the doctor-prescribed drug recommended for her lung cancer treatment. She received word, in an unsigned letter from the health plan administrator, that the state would not cover the drug to help extend her life, but it would pay for other drugs and the help of a doctor to kill her.

"To say to someone, we'll pay for you to die, but not pay for you to live, it's cruel," Wagner told the *Eugene Register-Guard*. "I get angry. Who do they think they are?"[52]

"We can't cover everything for everyone," a spokesman for Oregon's Division of Medical Assistance Programs told the *Register-Guard*. "Taxpayer dollars are limited for publicly funded programs. We try to come up with policies that provide the most good for the most people."[53]

Cutting costs by rationing care and ending lives has also been suggested in Vermont, a state which adopted a single-payer health care plan in May 2011. The owner of the *Addison County Independent* relayed the views of Stephen Kimbell, commissioner of Vermont's department of Banking, Insurance, Securities and Health Care Administration:

> Money must also be saved in services delivered to people with chronic diseases and those who frequently use emergency rooms, he [Kimbell] said; two areas in which the community at large must help play an important role.
> Passing a law that allows physicians to help end a patient's life under very controlled circumstances, known as "death with dignity," is one such measure that could help (an effort was tried this pass [sic] session but postponed until next year).
> Another is approving some type of rationing measures, as Oregon has done, that help control health care costs.[54]

Bio-ethics watchdog Wesley Smith observed, "If people think that rationing and assisted suicide aren't going to go hand in hand with a financial system [of] centralized control with real constraints on spending, I'm sorry, it's not alarmism; it's facts on the ground. It's already beginning to happen."⁵⁵

Vermont's neighbor, Massachusetts, adopted a government-run health plan in 2006, on which some parts of the federal health care overhaul were modeled. As more people, previously uninsured, entered the system without a proportionate increase in doctors, wait times to see a primary-care doctor jumped to as many as 100 days by 2008, according to the *Boston Globe*.⁵⁶

In 2010, the Massachusetts Medical Society found "more than half of primary care practices closed to new patients, longer wait times to get appointments with primary and specialty physicians, and significant variations in physician acceptance of government and government-related insurance products."⁵⁷

Columnist Doug Bandow reported that 20 percent of adults say they are having a hard time finding a doctor.⁵⁸ One resident said, "Before I was uninsured and couldn't see a doctor. Then I made the sacrifice to buy insurance, but I still can't find a doctor who will see me. So I still don't get to see a doctor, but it's costing me more now."⁵⁹

Many of those who are unable to see a doctor wind up in emergency rooms instead. The *Boston Globe* reported in April 2009 that "thousands of newly insured Massachusetts residents are relying on emergency rooms for routine medical care, an expensive habit that drives up health care costs and thwarts a major goal of the state's first in the nation health insurance law."⁶⁰

One solution proposed in the Massachusetts legislature has been to force doctors to see Medicaid patients on pain of the loss of their license to practice medicine.⁶¹ If doctors are unwilling to provide care for patients on whom they lose money, the solution for at least one Bay State legislator was to coerce them to do so.

State Treasurer Timothy P. Cahill has called the Massachusetts program a "fiscal train wreck." He wrote in the *Wall Street Journal* that four years after the program began, with a projected taxpayer expense of $88 million, total costs had jumped to $4 billion.⁶²

Those cost overruns have brought efforts to impose cost controls which, if successful, will mean rationing, as the Beacon Hill Institute warned: "Controlling costs will translate into capping services provided by physicians and other caregivers. These are, in effect, price controls that will dampen the incentive to provide services and lead to longer wait times and the rationing of healthcare."[63]

And that's what the future holds for the nation when the health care law, with its "rate-cutting machine," the Independent Payment Advisory Board, is fully implemented.

CHAPTER 3

RATIONCARE AT HOME

Those who worry that the new health care law will bring rationing to American medicine have sound reason for concern. And it's not just because the 2,801-page law sharply reduces Medicare payments to doctors by $575 billion and insulates those cuts from political pressure by creating the Independent Payment Advisory Board as an enforcement mechanism.

Other signals at the federal level—in both personnel and policy—point to a readiness to cut costs by reducing care. That predisposition to ration health care will heavily influence how the health law is administered. Donald Berwick, the man President Obama named in a 2010 recess appointment to head the Centers for Medicare and Medicaid Services (CMS), has made it plain that he thinks rationing is inevitable.

Berwick, who stepped down from his post on December 2, 2011, told the magazine *Biotechnology Healthcare* in 2009 that rationing was a *fait accompli*: "The decision is not whether or not we will ration care—the decision is whether we will ration with our eyes open. And right now, we are doing it blindly."[64]

Another Obama appointee to the Social Security Advisory Board, Henry Aaron, supports both rationing and IPAB. Aaron argued in a 1990 *Science* article that America must move toward health care rationing. Technology, with its abundance of medical innovations, "shows little sign of abating," Aaron wrote, "therefore the U.S. will have to ration care to slow the growth of health care spending."[65]

Aaron joined more than a dozen economists in November 2009 to urge President Obama to strengthen "the capacity of health reform to control the growth of spending."[66] More recently, he has come out against the repeal of IPAB, arguing instead that the board's role should be expanded to allow it to make cost-cutting recommendations not just for payments to doctors, but also to hospitals and clinical labs, both of which are off-limits to IPAB until 2020 and 2016, respectively.[67]

Several recent federal health care policy decisions also illustrate how cost and efficacy considerations are entering into the decision matrix. Federal law prohibits Medicare from denying treatment based solely on cost, but a Centers for Medicare and Medicaid Services internal email released through a Freedom of Information Act lawsuit filed by Judicial Watch includes reference to the cost and benefit of a treatment under review.

The Centers for Medicare and Medicaid Services launched a controversial review in 2010 of Provenge, a Food and Drug Administration (FDA)-approved treatment for prostate cancer that costs $93,000 per year per patient. William D. Rogers, Director of the CMS Physicians Regulatory Issues Team, emailed Louis B. Jacques, CMS Director of Coverage Analysis Group, on June 8, 2010:

> We discussed this on the last CMD [Contract Medical Director] call. $93,000 per treatment adds four months to life, 27,000 patients a year $2.6 billion dollars a year.[68]

Judicial Watch president Tom Fitton reports that the Obama

administration denies that the Provenge review was done because of the treatment's cost. Under pressure from both care providers and the public, CMS announced on June 30, 2011, that it will pay for Provenge treatments of prostate cancer.

PUTTING COST ABOVE TREATMENT

In November 2011, the federal government weighed in against the use of a breast cancer treatment when the FDA lifted its approval of Avastin, a drug used to treat advanced breast cancer. A preliminary FDA advisory panel ruled in 2010 against the drug's use for advanced breast cancer, prompting the *Wall Street Journal* to call that action "an American precedent for the medical central planning of ObamaCare."[69] The *Journal* said the advisory panel's recommendation "betrays a bias that puts costs above treatment" and noted that one panel member said of her anti-Avastin vote, "We aren't supposed to talk about cost, but that's another issue."

In 2009, the federal Preventive Services Task Force changed longstanding recommendations on mammograms, recommending that women between 50 and 74 get them every other year and that they be skipped altogether for women in their forties. Public uproar followed the panel's recommendations, which some saw as a preview of coming attractions as the government employs "comparative effectiveness research" to evaluate treatments.

In revising its mammogram recommendations, the task force made a "financial calculation," according to health policy expert Sally Pipes, president of the Pacific Research Institute. The task force concluded that while one woman would be spared for every 1,900 screenings of women in their forties, it would take 1,300 screenings to spare one woman in her fifties, and 377 screenings for women in their sixties. Mammograms then, become more cost effective as women grow older.

"But does that mean that women in their forties shouldn't get mammograms?" asks Pipes. "What if the life saved is yours— or your mother's, daughter's, or sister's?... Do we really want bureaucrats deciding whose life is worth saving?"[70] It's worth noting that under the new health care law, the federal Preventive Services Task Force has the job of determining coverage for preventive services.[71]

The task force again stirred up controversy and concern over health care rationing in October 2011 when it issued a draft recommendation that physically healthy men should not be given the PSA blood test, which screens for prostate cancer. The task force ruling came, the *New York Times* reported, because "the test does not save lives over all and often leads to more tests and treatments that needlessly cause pain, impotence and incontinence in many...."[72]

But Dr. Deepak Kapoor, the head of Advanced Urology Centers of New York, the largest urology group practice in the nation, said, "Removing PSA blood tests would be an extremely negative step for men's health." Kapoor claimed that, "Because of early detection efforts, the death rate from prostate cancer has decreased 38% (from almost 40 per 100,000 men in 1992 to fewer than 25 per 100,000 in 2007). During this interval, the incidence of prostate cancer has been virtually flat."[73]

At least two insurers, Aetna and Kaiser Permanente, said they were undecided if they would still pay for the PSA test in the wake of the task force decision.

"This rationing may not be as overt as one sees in socialized systems like the United Kingdom, but it still holds the potential to restrict a patient's ability to receive the care they desire," Texas Public Policy Foundation policy analyst Spencer Harris wrote. "A patient's health care decisions should not be determined by the recommendations of any federal board, no matter how distant."[74]

Dr. Michael Koch, chairman of the urology department at the Indiana University School of Medicine, called the task force's recommendation "almost insulting to the patient. It's paternalistic...."[75]

It also foreshadows the rationing that will come to America under the new healthcare law, with its "automatic policies and depoliticized commissions" of which IPAB, as former White House budget chief Peter Orszag put it, is, "Perhaps the most dramatic example...."

CUTTING MEDICARE

Author Peter Ferrara, a Harvard-trained attorney who serves as general counsel of the American Civil Rights Union, believes that the Patient Protection and Affordable Care Act "provides for a comprehensive system of government rationing of health care"[76] that is achieved via massive cuts to Medicare funding, financial incentives that steer care away from the sick and the old, reliance on "comparative effectiveness research," and more.

Medicare, the federal insurance program established by Congress in 1965, serves about 15 percent of the U.S. population. Some 47.5 million people were on Medicare in 2010 (39.6 million aged 65 and older and 7.9 million disabled). Total Medicare spending in 2010 was $523 billion, with income of just $486 billion ($37 billion below expense).[77]

Those numbers are going to have to change under the new health law. It cuts some $575 billion from Medicare between 2010 and 2019, according to Richard Foster, the chief actuary for the Centers for Medicare and Medicaid Services.[78] But the first decade cuts to Medicare are actually $800 billion when measured from 2014, the first year the law is fully implemented. And the cuts grow from there, totaling $2.9 trillion over the first two decades of actual implementation.[79]

Galen Institute president Grace-Marie Turner told a House Budget Committee hearing in July 2011 that if the cuts already in the law take place, "seniors could face long waits for appointments and treatments, and many would be forced to wait in line in over-crowded emergency rooms to get care, just as Medicaid patients do throughout the country today."[80]

Ferrara believes that the Medicare cuts in the Affordable Care Act "would create havoc and chaos in health care for seniors."[81] He cites Richard Foster, the CMS chief actuary, who believes that 15 percent of health care professionals serving the elderly may drop out due to Medicare cuts. Those who think that health care rationing is not on its way, courtesy of the Affordable Care Act, may want to contemplate Foster's warning:

> Thus, providers for whom Medicare constitutes a

substantive portion of their business could find it difficult to remain profitable and, absent legislative intervention, might end their participation in the program (possibly jeopardizing access to care for beneficiaries). Simulations by the Office of the Actuary suggest that roughly 15 percent of Part A providers would become unprofitable within the 10-year projection period as a result of the productivity adjustments.[82]

If 15 percent of Medicare providers become unprofitable and, presumably, go out of business, the elderly will find themselves waiting longer for care or going without. As Ferrara puts it, "If the government is not going to pay, then seniors are not going to get the health services, treatment and care they expect."[83]

That is already happening. A Mayo Clinic near Phoenix, Arizona, announced in late 2009 that it will no longer accept Medicare patients and would require existing patients to pay cash to see their doctors. The change affected some 3,000 Medicare patients, according to a Mayo spokesman, who said Mayo, nationwide, lost $840 million on Medicare in 2008.[84]

FEWER HEALTH CARE OPTIONS

Aside from huge reductions in Medicare funding, the new health care law will likely lead to fewer insurance firms, doctors, and hospitals—and therefore fewer health care options for ordinary Americans. The Affordable Care Act does this, for example, by making it more difficult for new insurance firms to compete. It prescribes a limit to how much can be spent on marketing, often a large cost for firms seeking to enter new markets. The law also makes it more difficult for firms to distinguish themselves from other, more well-established competitors, since all health plans must conform to federal specifications.

Insurance firms must also accept applicants without regard to pre-existing conditions, and premiums cannot be adjusted based on an individual applicant's health. Those two requirements, "guaranteed issue" and "community rating," will have a number of perverse effects, not the least of which will be to encourage "free-riders"—individuals who, knowing they cannot be refused, sign up for insurance coverage only when a need for health care arises.

Ferrara suggests that the increased financial exposure stemming from both guaranteed issue and community rating will encourage insurance firms to migrate to provider networks that are less likely to serve those who are most sick. Instead, they will seek to insure the young and healthy. He quotes John Goodman, president of the National Center for Policy Analysis, and Gerald Musgrave, who have written, "The easiest way [for insurers] to keep costs down is to enroll only the healthy. And the easiest way to do that is not to have the doctors and facilities sick people want."[85]

Ferrara acknowledges that the law may not allow insurers to so transparently avoid the financial risk imposed by guaranteed issue and community rating but insists that "it is clear that networks will be narrowed to attract or repel some classes of patients to drive better economics, reducing patient choice."[86]

The new law also creates a system to track Medicare expenditures by doctor and introduces a means by which doctors may be penalized for spending too many Medicare treatment dollars. That kind of pressure is prompting doctors to exit their individual or group practices or to become salaried employees at hospitals or clinics. What that means for patients is less care and less caring since, as Ferrara points out, "Salaried doctors are unlikely to be willing to be on call 24 hours a day, to develop long-term relationships that can lead to greater familiarity with patients' conditions, and to be advocates for their patients against insurers and hospital administrators who place a higher emphasis on limiting spending than relieving pain or finding a cure."[87]

Another way in which the new law limits access to health care is by shutting down the construction of new physician-owned hospitals. The advocacy group, Physicians Hospital of America (PHA), announced in January 2011 that construction was forced to stop at 45 doctor-owned hospitals nationwide.[88] This is due to a provision in the health care law that "effectively bans new physician-owned hospitals (POHs) from starting up, and … keeps existing ones from expanding," according to Heartland Institute writer Kenneth Artz.[89] A PHA survey found that 55 percent of physician-owned hospitals nationwide would expand, investing $1.8 billion on construction and creating 6,300 full time health care jobs, if not for the limitation imposed by the Affordable Care Act.[90]

Ferrara predicts that the pressures placed upon the health care industry by the health law will lead to consolidation and "a small number of insurers, hospital chains, and clinic chains with much greater power to implement rationing, and government policies favoring more such rationing than is currently possible. Consumers will be left with little choice or power."[91]

And that's before we factor in the sweeping power of the Independent Payment Advisory Board to restructure health care and impose *de facto* rationing.

CHAPTER 4

AMERICA'S NEW "RATIONING BOARD"

The authors of Public Law 111–148, the "Patient Protection and Affordable Care Act," named it the Independent Payment Advisory Board, or IPAB. But in the months since President Obama's April 13, 2011, speech on the deficit brought IPAB to wider public attention,[92] it has been called a great many other things.

"The real death panel,"[93] "a rationing board,"[94] "RationCare,"[95] "the royal road to socialism,"[96] and "a Beltway acronym for subverting the deliberative process"[97] are just a few of the colorful reproaches invented for IPAB.

Its advocates, by contrast, shower IPAB with terms of endearment. Former White House budget chief Peter Orszag calls it a "very promising structure," while Brookings Institution economist Henry Aaron hails IPAB as "Congress' 'Good Deed'" and an exercise of legislative "statesmanship."

Whatever the label, all agree that IPAB is, first and foremost, a potent mechanism to reduce Medicare spending while shielded from public and political pressure. For that it is praised and pilloried.

Sen. Tom Coburn (R-OK) offers a clear summary of the case against IPAB:

> There are virtually no checks on the panel, since its members are not answerable to voters and its recommendations cannot be challenged in court. Because the panel is barred from examining common-sense changes like Medicare beneficiary premiums, cost-sharing, or benefit design, many expect that in efforts to control spending, the panel will limit patient access to medical care.[98]

IPAB is, as its name declares, truly "independent." It is not subject to the normal rules which govern other federal commissions requiring public notice, the opportunity for public comment, and public review. And if an American citizen disagrees with the implementation of an IPAB recommendation, he or she has no legal recourse. As the law states, "There shall be no administrative judicial review…."[99]

HARD TO PULL THE PLUG

The law makes it very hard for Congress to defund IPAB. The Board's annual budget is already appropriated in the health care law by a "permanent mechanism" that "appropriates (and transfers from the Medicare Trust Funds) $15 million for FY 2012, with automatic subsequent appropriations" indexed for inflation thereafter.[100]

Support exists for measures introduced in the House and Senate to repeal IPAB. Passage in the House seems assured, as a majority of 218 members have already co-sponsored a bill to repeal it. Co-sponsors include several liberals who originally supported the health care law, among them Rep. Pete Stark and Rep. Barney Franks. A similar repeal measure in the Senate, the "Health Care Bureaucrats Elimination Act," has 32 co-sponsors.[101]

Some 270 health care groups that represent "doctors, other healthcare providers, employers, drug and medical device manufacturers and some disease-specific advocates" called in June 2011 for IPAB's repeal.[102] The Healthcare Leadership Council (HLC) has joined in the call, stating in a letter that "HLC is concerned about rationing of care as a result of IPAB actions."[103] Other groups calling for repeal include the American Hospital Association, the Pharmaceutical Research and Manufacturers of America, and two large nursing home associations, the American Health Care Association and the American Association of Homes and Services for the Aging.[104]

IPAB's insulation from the courts, Congress, and the public make it a stand-alone law-making body—and a mockery of the system of separated powers established in the U.S. Constitution. Wesley J. Smith calls it a "super legislature" and the "cornerstone... of a bureaucratic state." He warns that "when you give that bureaucracy the power of legislation so that it can potentially even overcome a presidential veto ... then you have changed the very nature of governance in the United States of America."[105]

In passing this law, Congress gave a panel of 15 people appointed by the president the authority to make law. That's why the Goldwater Institute, an Arizona think tank, has challenged IPAB in court. The group's litigation director, Clint Bolick, says, "No possible reading of the Constitution supports the idea of an unelected, standalone federal board that's untouchable by both Congress and the courts."[106]

In testimony to Congress, Goldwater Institute attorney Diane Cohen blasted the health care law's creation of IPAB as "the most sweeping delegation of congressional authority in history...."[107]

Despite the frequent use of the word "recommendations" to describe IPAB proposals, Cohen told the *Weekly Standard* that IPAB is

> not making recommendations to Congress. They're really going to be passing law. The statute actually

calls it "law" throughout the Patient Protection and Affordable Care Act. Congress doesn't have to pass them; the president doesn't have to sign them. So it's taking over a historically congressional responsibility and duty....[108]

It's also giving political cover to elected members of Congress who can wash their hands of any responsibility when IPAB issues painful cuts to payments or procedures. Which is why, as observed earlier, IPAB earns such high marks from government health care reform advocates like Orszag and Daschle.

IPAB's 15 members are appointed by the president and confirmed by the Senate to serve staggered six-year terms. The qualifications for appointment include "expertise in health finance and economics, actuarial science, health facility management, health plans and integrated delivery systems...."[109] Board members cannot have other employment and are paid $163,500 a year. Beyond the appointed board members, there are three *ex officio* non-voting members: the Secretary of Health and Human Services (HHS), the Administrator of the Centers for Medicare and Medicaid Services (CMA), and the Administrator of the Health Resources and Services Administration (HRSA).

The law charges IPAB with the responsibility of submitting annual proposals to Congress and the president, beginning in 2014, on how to stem Medicare spending if it is growing too fast. Those recommendations are law unless Congress rejects them with a majority vote in the House, and a 60-vote supermajority in the Senate, and produces an alternative plan to reach spending reduction targets that is signed by the President. The law does prohibit IPAB from issuing recommendations that would raise taxes, alter benefits, or ration care. However, health policy expert Sally Pipes believes that "it's almost certain that IPAB proposals will lead to these outcomes indirectly."[110]

DE FACTO RATIONING

It's hard to imagine any other outcome than *de facto* rationing from IPAB price controls. As payments decline, doctors will be forced to drop out of Medicare or withhold some medical services—and that will leave Medicare patients standing in line or going without.

Not all of Medicare is subject to IPAB cuts. The law exempts hospitals and hospices until 2020, as well as clinical labs until 2016.[111] What remains for IPAB's budget knife is "Medicare Advantage, the Part D prescription drug program; skilled nursing facility, home health, dialysis, ambulance and ambulatory surgical center services; and durable medical equipment."[112]

It's quite likely that IPAB will "look to MA [Medicare Advantage] for a big chunk of the spending reductions it must find beginning in 2014 if Medicare cost growth exceeds the targeted rate each year," according to *Medicare Advantage News*.[113] Medicare Advantage is a partially private program which gives seniors more health care options. The number of MA enrollees has doubled since 2003 to about 11 million people, or 22 percent of Medicare beneficiaries.[114] Those numbers may decline in coming years as reductions in federal payments take effect. The federal subsidy to MA was frozen in 2011 under the health care law and will decline in future years, affecting seniors who utilize this popular option.

SEBELIUS: "HUGE REDUCTIONS IN CARE"

Health and Human Services Secretary Kathleen Sebelius vigorously defends IPAB, saying the law "expressly" prohibits IPAB from recommendations to ration care. But Sebelius had to concede that payment cuts would lead to a reduction in services when pressed by Rep. Joe Pitts (R-PA) at a House hearing. As reported in *The Weekly Standard*, Pitts asked Sebelius whether seniors would be affected by IPAB recommendations to reduce payments for dialysis services.

> "If Congress accepted the recommendations and made the decision that cuts in dialysis were appropriate," Sebelius replied, "I assume there could be some providers who would decide that would not be a service they would any longer deliver, the same

way they do with insurance providers each and every day."

"Would that mean some seniors have to wait longer for dialysis?" Pitts asked.

"Mr. Chairman, as you know, any cut in services, certainly cost shifting to beneficiaries, could mean huge reductions in care that seniors would have the opportunity to receive," said Sebelius.[115]

It is bad enough that IPAB payment reductions will reduce needed health care for seniors; some of its proponents want it to do even more to cut spending and give it authority over private health care spending as well.

That may happen even without altering IPAB's legal charter if, as health policy expert Peter Ferrara predicts, Medicare payment policy is "copied by private insurers, spreading the impact throughout the entire health care system."[116]

Both President Barack Obama's deficit reduction plan and his budget commission have proposed added authority for the IPAB, but the details about those enhanced powers remain unknown, as noted by Brookings Institution scholar Henry Aaron.[117]

MORE POWER TO IPAB

In his April 2011 deficit speech, President Barack Obama spoke of

> strengthening an independent commission of doctors, nurses, medical experts and consumers who will look at all the evidence and recommend the best ways to reduce unnecessary spending while protecting access to the services seniors need.[118]

The President claimed in his speech that the Affordable Care Act will achieve savings of $1.5 trillion by 2033. But, he added, "if we're wrong, and Medicare costs rise faster than we expect," strengthening IPAB will give it "the authority to make additional savings by further improving Medicare."[119]

The President has proposed squeezing Medicare even

more, suggesting that IPAB "be directed to limit Medicare cost growth per beneficiary to GDP growth per capita plus 0.5 percent beginning in 2018,"[120] instead of the one percent above GDP growth presently called for in the health care law. He has also floated the idea of giving "IPAB additional enforcement mechanisms such as an automatic sequester"[121] of congressional appropriations.

As Grace-Marie Turner, president of the Galen Institute, said in testimony to Congress, "It is far from clear where the constitutional authority is for a board of appointees housed in the Executive Branch to usurp the power of Congress by sequestering funds if Congress were to decide to override its rulings."[122]

Former Senate Majority leader Tom Daschle told the *New York Times*, one month after the health care law's passage, that IPAB's authority should grow to deal with the world of private health insurance. Otherwise, lowered Medicare reimbursements to doctors will lead doctors to try to make up for their lost income through private insurance.[123]

That kind of cost-shifting is a huge concern. One study found that private insurance costs are already 22 percent higher due to insufficient payments through Medicare and Medicaid that are shifted to the private sector.[124]

For supporters of the new health law, a solution to cost-shifting is to give IPAB authority over private insurance rates as well. Writing in the *New England Journal of Medicine*, health law expert Timothy S. Jost acknowledges that "health care providers may well abandon Medicare" due to underpayments to doctors. The solution to the problem, he suggests, may be to give IPAB authority over all health insurance rates, public and private:

> In the long run, Congress may not be able to cap Medicare expenditures without addressing private expenditures as well. If the IPAB opens the door to rate setting for all payers, it may well be the most revolutionary innovation of the ACA.[125]

The revolution—or something close to it—may have already

taken place. An analysis by the National Right to Life Committee argues that the law already gives IPAB authority to issue mandates that must be followed by private insurers as well.

The new health care law requires IPAB to submit recommendations to Congress, not just for Medicare payment reductions, but also for private health care spending in the nation at large. Those latter recommendations are said to be advisory, but the Powell Center for Medical Ethics at the National Right to Life Committee thinks otherwise.

Starting in 2015, IPAB is required by the law to "submit to Congress and the President recommendations to slow the growth in national health expenditures [outside of Medicare] … while preserving or enhancing quality of care…."[126]

The first thing to know is that, as the Kaiser Health Institute reports, "There are no constraints on the scope of what IPAB can include in its advisory recommendations"[127] to put the brakes on health care spending. The second is that, as the NRLC argues, these recommendations may not, in fact, be merely "advisory."

A report on the Powell Center's website states:[128]

> An 18-member "Independent Payment Advisory Board" is given the duty, on January 15, 2015, and every two years thereafter, with regard to private (not just governmentally funded) health care, to make "recommendations to slow the growth in national health expenditures" below the rate of medical inflation.[129]
>
> The Commission's recommendations are to be ones "that the Secretary [of Health and Human Services] or other Federal agencies can implement administratively."[130] In turn, the Secretary of Health and Human Services is empowered to impose "quality and efficiency" measures on hospitals, requiring them to report on their compliance with them.[131] Doctors will have to comply with such quality measures in order to be able to contract with any qualified insurance plan.[132]
>
> Basically, doctors, hospitals, and other health care providers will be told by Washington just what

diagnostic tests and medical care are considered to meet "quality and efficiency" standards—not only for federally funded programs like Medicare, but also for health care paid for by private citizens and their nongovernmental health insurance.

In effect, there will be one uniform national standard of care established by Washington bureaucrats and set with a view to limiting what private citizens are allowed to spend on saving their own lives.

It is stunning to think that an unaccountable, unelected federal board may have been empowered by the new health care law to dictate the details of health care spending in the private American economy. But the legal analysis above suggests it has.

"WE'RE GOING TO LET YOU DIE"

Those who doubt that such a scenario could even be contemplated, let alone made law in America, should ponder the following remarks delivered by Clinton Administration Labor Secretary Robert Reich to an audience at the University of California, Berkeley, on September 9, 2007. Reich offered a candid admission that health care reform would limit health care options for all of us. He said that an "honest" presidential candidate would tell Americans that health care reform would mean young people will pay more, the elderly will die sooner, and medical innovation will suffer. Such a presidential candidate, according to Reich, would tell Americans the following:

> I would like to be president. Let me tell you a few things on health care.... What I am going to do is I am going to try to reorganize [American health care] to make it more amendable to treating sick people but that means you, particularly you young people, particularly you young healthy people, you're going to have to pay more.
>
> And, by the way ... if you're very old, we're not going to give you all that technology and all those

drugs for the last couple of years of your life to keep you maybe going for another couple of months. It's too expensive. So we're going to let you die.

Also, I'm going to use the bargaining leverage of the federal government in terms of Medicare, Medicaid ... to force drug companies and insurance companies and medical suppliers to reduce their costs, but that means less innovation and that means less new products and less new drugs on the market, which means you are probably not going to live that much longer than your parents.[133]

And that straight talk brings us to the topic of "death panels."

CHAPTER 5

HEALTH CARE IN A POST-CHRISTIAN WORLD

Former Alaska governor Sarah Palin outraged advocates of government health care reform when she charged, in August 2009, that a provision in pending health care legislation would introduce a "death panel" into American medicine. In her sharply worded blast, Palin wrote:

> [G]overnment health care will not reduce the cost; it will simply refuse to pay the cost. And who will suffer the most when they ration care? The sick, the elderly, and the disabled, of course. The America I know and love is not one in which my parents or my baby with Down Syndrome will have to stand in front of Obama's "death panel" so his bureaucrats can decide, based on a subjective judgment of their "level of productivity in society," whether they are worthy of health care. Such a system is downright evil.[134]

Her Facebook post referenced a provision to pay doctors to counsel elderly patients about living wills, advance directives, and end-of-life care options. That language was soon removed from the health care bill. A similar provision inserted into proposed Medicare regulations at the end of 2009 was also pulled after it became public.[135]

Palin's thoughts provoked rebukes from many. *The New York Times* labeled the "death panel" claim a "stubborn, but false rumor"[136] and then-*Newsweek* editor Jon Meacham called it "a lie crafted to foment opposition to the president's push for reform."[137]

"KILLING GRANNY"

But under the headline, "The Case for Killing Granny," Meacham's *Newsweek* colleague Evan Thomas declared that, while it is "political anathema" to talk about health care rationing for seniors, "the need to spend less money on the elderly at the end of life is the elephant in the room in the health-reform debate."[138]

Straight talk like that helps explain why Palin's "death panel" post made the impact it did. Despite official denials, there is enough pro-rationing chatter in American culture to raise public anxiety. *The New York Times* itself came out for health care rationing in 2010, arguing,

> without curtailing the use of unnecessary, overly costly and even dangerous new technologies and surgical procedures, there is little hope of restraining the relentless rise in health care costs.[139]

Former Colorado Governor Richard Lamm claimed in 2011 that rationing could fix health care. Lamm thinks seniors should lower their "unrealistic expectations" for quality health care and asserted, "Rationing is the price an aging society must pay to prevent health care from crowding out all other public needs."[140]

That is not comforting for people who are already or soon-to-be retired. Alarm over the prospect of government-mandated health care rationing only grows when Congress creates a powerful, free-standing, independent health care control board like IPAB. One empowered to issue edicts which are beyond appeal or judicial review.

Yes, the law prohibits IPAB from instituting health care rationing but, as noted earlier, rationing will result when IPAB's Medicare payment reduction "recommendations" are issued and become law. Doctors will drop out of Medicare, leave medicine, or withhold unfunded or underfunded procedures. And sometimes death will result.

It has already happened. Two people waiting for organ transplants in Arizona died after the state Health Care Cost Containment System put a halt to seven types of organ transplants. The system made the decision after the state legislature, faced with a severe budget shortfall, cut Medicaid funding in 2010.[141]

Wesley Smith observes that "no private insurance company would dare unilaterally deny a previously qualified patient life-saving surgery, as Arizona did. Only government can get away with something like that."[142] More of the same is what could be just ahead once IPAB, with its power to limit Medicare spending, begins issuing recommendations in 2014.

ETHICAL SHIFT

The Independent Payment Advisory Board comes at a time of transformation in American medical ethics. "We're in the midst of a shift in healthcare ethics, medical ethics, away from a sanctity-of-life, Hippocratic value system into a much more utilitarian system—even a consumer-oriented system," says Smith.[143]

It's a shift, say Chuck Colson and Nancy Pearcey, from a culture of life to "what John Paul II called a 'culture of death,' a naturalistic ethic sweeping across the entire spectrum, from the unborn to the old and infirm, from the deformed and disabled to the weak and defenseless."[144]

The shift has been going on for a generation. Francis Schaeffer said in 1982 that the "medical profession has radically changed." He recalled the words of Dr. C. Everett Koop, a celebrated pediatric surgeon who served as U.S. Surgeon General under President Reagan: "When I graduated from medical school [1941], the idea was, 'How can I save this life?' But for a great number of the medical students now, it's not, 'How can I save this life?' but 'Should I save this life?'"

Doctors and bioethicists now have the power, Smith notes, "to say, 'No,' to wanted, and I emphasize, wanted, life-sustaining treatment based on a quality of life judgmentalism that is pernicious."

In 2006 a bioethics committee at Houston's St. Luke's Hospital ordered Andrea Clarke's life support removed, even though she was not unconscious and her family wanted her to continue receiving treatment. The order came, Smith has written, under "futile-care theory," which holds that "even if the patient can communicate that he or she wants life-sustaining treatment—it can be withheld anyway if the doctors and/or the ethics committee believe that the quality of the patient's life renders it not worth living."[145]

"DUTY TO DIE"

Some bioethicists now assert that people who are disabled, very ill, or at the end of life, have a "duty to die" rather than burden the family or state. University of Tennessee philosophy professor John Hardwig wrote in 1997:

> A duty to die is more likely when continuing to live will impose significant burdens—emotional burdens, extensive caregiving, destruction of life plans, and yes, financial hardship—on your family and loved ones.[146]

Hardwig, now retired, dismissed the idea that "God, the giver of life, forbids that anyone take her own life" and says that "there can be a duty to die when one would prefer to live."[147]

The "duty to die" has an influential champion in the United Kingdom, where well-known bio-ethicist Baroness Mary Warnock has held that people with Alzheimer's burden others and may have an obligation to die. Baroness Warnock told a

Church of Scotland magazine in 2008, "If you're demented, you're wasting people's lives—your family's lives—and you're wasting the resources of the National Health Service."[148]

Warnock proposed people draw up advanced directives while they still have their wits about them and assign a caregiver willing to euthanize them if they succumb to dementia. "I think that's the way the future will go, putting it rather brutally, you'd be licensing people to put others down," said Warnock.[149]

Baroness Warnock would have been right at home in ancient Greece or Rome, cultures where compassion for the sick and dying was a rare thing. Alvin J. Schmidt, author of *How Christianity Changed the World*, writes that Greek philosopher "Plato (427-347 B.C.) said that a poor man (usually a slave) who was no longer able to work because of sickness should be left to die."[150] Schmidt also cites Plautus (254-184 B.C.), a Roman philosopher who argued, "You do a beggar bad service by giving him food and drink; you lose what you give and prolong his life for more misery."[151]

The same attitude applied to the young. "Saving physically frail, unwanted children was an affront to the Romans. It violated their cultural norms," writes Schmidt. The first century Roman philosopher Seneca declared: "We drown children who at birth are weakly and abnormal."[152]

But all that changed with the coming of Christianity. "Prior to the coming of Christ, human life on this planet was exceedingly cheap. Life was expendable prior to Christianity's influence," write D. James Kennedy and Jerry Newcombe in their book, *What If Jesus Had Never Been Born?*[153] "Jesus Christ— He who said, 'Behold, I make all things new' (Revelation 21:5)— gave mankind a new perspective on the value of human life."

HEALTH CARE ROOTED IN CHRISTIANITY

While neither the Greeks nor the Romans built hospitals for the general public,[154] Christianity introduced "charity hospitals for the poor and indigent," Schmidt writes.[155] In fact, health care and hospitals are rooted in Christianity. It was Christianity that, in large part, gave rise to the West's long tradition of compassionate, sacrificial medical care. That tradition began with Jesus Christ, who brought healing to many during his earthly ministry and instructed His followers to do the same.

When plague struck Alexandria about 250 A.D., it was every man for himself among the pagans, according to the Christian bishop Dionysius. They "thrust aside anyone who began to be sick, and kept aloof even from their dearest friends, and cast the sufferers out upon the public roads half dead, and left them unburied, and treated them with utter contempt when they died."[156]

Christians did the opposite, as Dionysius reported:

> [V]ery many of our brethren, while in their exceeding love and brotherly kindness did not spare themselves, but kept by each other, and visited the sick without thought of their own peril, and ministered to them assiduously and treated them for their healing in Christ, died from time to time most joyfully … drawing upon themselves their neighbors' diseases, and willingly taking over to their own persons the burden of the sufferings of those around them.[157]

The Council of Nicea in 325 A.D. ordered that hospices be established in every cathedral city in Christendom.[158] St. Basil built the first hospital with beds about 369 A.D.[159] By the middle of the 6th century, hospitals were established in most of Christendom, east and west.[160] Compassion for the sick continued to expand and, Schmidt notes, there were some 37,000 Benedictine monasteries that cared for the ill by the mid-1500s.[161]

Christianity's influence did not stop there. Modern nursing owes much to Florence Nightingale, a 19th century nurse and nursing educator who, as Kennedy and Newcombe note, "received much of the inspiration for her work from Jesus Christ."[162] Henry Dunant, an evangelical Swiss banker and philanthropist, founded the International Red Cross in the mid-19th century. He did so out of a sense of calling from God.[163] The Red Cross has helped save millions of lives since its inception and, as Kennedy and Newcombe write, "[I]t was founded by an evangelical."[164]

But now Christian influence in health care is waning, and our post-Christian culture is returning to pagan attitudes toward human life. Instead of the ethic inspired by Jesus Christ, who told His followers to "... heal the sick" (Luke 9:2), bioethicists promote the "duty to die," and a utilitarian approach to life is taking hold in American health care. Add to that new ethic a government takeover of health care featuring an unaccountable payment board with power to determine health care spending decisions for seniors, and, if some of its advocates get their wish, for all Americans.

Difficult days may be ahead—especially for the weak and elderly. Unless, of course, Americans stand up and say no to government by unaccountable experts and demand that Congress repeal the Independent Payment Advisory Board.

"IT'S UP TO US"

But that is just a start. The centralization of American health care won't be stopped unless the Patient Protection and Affordable Care Act is overturned in *toto*—whether by the U.S. Supreme Court, by our elected representatives in Washington, or by the American public next November.

"The American people get to decide," says Wesley Smith. "Do we want centralized health care or do we not? ... The good thing is it's up to us."[165]

America is in the midst of a conflict over competing worldviews. The authors of a critical review of the health care law note that the 2009-2010 battle in Congress over health care legislation "was never about policy, but rather a paternalistic ideology at odds with our historic commitment to individual liberty, limited government and entrepreneurial dynamism."[166]

That is certainly true, but the conflict goes even deeper. We are now divided between a health care ethic grounded in the Christian moral tradition and a utilitarian approach to health care, one in which a patient's worth to society figures heavily into the care he or she receives. And that fundamental ethical divide will continue, whatever the electoral outcome.

That is why, for Christians, our duty is not done, however November's elections turn out. Yes, we must indeed pray, be educated, talk with our neighbors, support godly candidates, and vote.

But that's not all. If we know Christ, we ought also to bear witness to the Gospel by our lips and by our lives. It is the influence of the Gospel, wielded in one-on-one encounters and through other means as well, that will unleash the same dynamic that once before transformed a pagan culture of death. It happened before. It can happen again. As C.S. Lewis once said, "He who converts his neighbour has performed the most practical Christian-political act of all."[167]

ENDNOTES

1   Robert Rector, "Strange Facts about America's 'Poor,'" *National Review*, September 13, 2011.http://www.nationalreview.com/corner/277040/strange-facts-about-america-s-poor-robert-rector.
2   Altarum Institute press release, "Health Sector Has 'Quiet' Month: Price, Spending, Employment Growth All Tick Down," MarketWatch.com, Dec. 8, 2011. http://www.marketwatch.com/story/health-sector-has-quiet-month-price-spending-employment-growth-all-tick-down-2011-12-08.
3   Peter Ferrara, *The Obamacare Disaster: An Appraisal of the Patient Protection and Affordable Care Act* (Chicago: The Heartland Institute, 2010, Kindle Edition).
4   The National Right to Life Committee (NRLC) explained in an Oct. 6, 2011, letter to members of the U.S. House of Representatives that the Patient Protection and Affordable Care Act "... contained multiple provisions that provide authorizations for subsidies for abortion, both implicit and explicit, and also multiple provisions that opened doors to abortion-expanding administrative actions." In testimony to Congress, NRLC legislative director Douglas Johnson described the Executive Order issued by President Obama to prohibit abortion funding in the health care law as a "hollow political construct—or, as described by the president of the Planned Parenthood Federation of America, 'a symbolic gesture.'"
5   A CNN poll taken March 19-21, 2010, just as the "Patient Protection and Affordable Care Act" won final passage in Congress, found 59 percent of Americans opposed the health care legislation. See CNN Opinion Research Poll at http://i2.cdn.turner.com/cnn/2010/images/03/22/rel5a.pdf.
6   Grace-Marie Turner; James C. Capretta; Thomas P. Miller; Robert E. Moffit, *Why Obamacare Is Wrong for America: How the New Health Care Law Drives Up Costs, Puts Government in Charge of Your Decisions, and Threatens Your Constitutional Rights* (City: Harper Collins, Inc., 2011), p. 21.
7   Ibid., p. 23.
8   Ibid., p. 47.
9   Ibid., p. 11.
10   Douglas Holtz-Eakin, "Medicare's Future: An Examination of the Independent Payment Advisory Board, Testimony before the United States House of Representatives Committee on the Budget," July 23, 2011, p. 2.

11	218 House members listed as co-sponsors of H.R. 452, the Medicare Decisions Accountability Act of 2011, as of Dec. 7, 2011. See http://thomas.loc.gov/home/thomas.php.
12	Douglas Holtz-Eakin, "Medicare's Future: An Examination of the Independent Payment Advisory Board, Testimony before the United States House of Representatives Committee on the Budget," July 23, 2011, p. 4.
13	"Will Obama Make Recess Appointments to Controversial IPAB?" Robert Powell Center for Medical Ethics at the National Right to Life Committee, June 29, 2011. http://powellcenterformedicalethics.blogspot.com/.
14	Bill Frist & John Breaux, "Keep Medicare in Congress' Hands," Politico.com, March 19, 2010. http://dyn.politico.com/members/forums/thread.cfm?catid=1&subcatid=4&threadid=3818397&sort=0.
15	Matthew Boyle, "'Real death panels' set to face heat in Congress, courts," *The Daily Caller*, March 22, 2011. http://dailycaller.com/2011/03/22/real-death-panels-set-to-face-heat-in-congress-courts/.
16	"Statement of Congressman Pete Stark Supporting Health Care Reform," March 21, 2010. http://www.stark.house.gov/index.php?option=com_content&view=article&id=1534:statement-of-congressman-pete-stark-supporting-health-care-reform&catid=67:floor-statements-2010-&Itemid=84.
17	Peter Orszag, "Too Much of a Good Thing: Why we need less democracy," *The New Republic*, September 14, 2011. http://www.tnr.com/article/politics/magazine/94940/peter-orszag-democracy.
18	The Federalist No. 51, "The Structure of the Government Must Furnish the Proper Checks and Balances Between the Different Departments." http://www.constitution.org/fed/federa51.htm.
19	M. E. Bradford, *A Worthy Company* (Marlborough, NH : Plymouth Rock Foundation, 1982), p. 147. Quoted in Jerry Newcombe, D. Min., *Answers from the Founding Fathers*, (Fort Lauderdale, FL: Truth in Action Ministries, 2011), p. 136.
20	Thomas Jefferson, Letter to Joseph C. Cabell, 2 Feb. 1816; *Works*, VI, 541, Caroline Thomas Harnsberger, ed., *Treasury of Presidential Quotations* (Chicago: Follett Publishing Company, 1964), p. 122. Quoted in Jerry Newcombe, D. Min., *Answers from the Founding Fathers*, (Fort Lauderdale, FL: Truth in Action Ministries, 2011), p. 134.
21	Catherine Drinker Bowen, *Miracle at Philadelphia: The Story of the Constitutional Convention May to September 1787* (Boston et al.: An Atlantic Monthly Press Book, a division of Little, Brown and Company, 1966/1986), p. 61. Quoted in Jerry Newcombe, D. Min., *Answers from the Founding Fathers*, (Fort Lauderdale, FL: Truth in Action Ministries, 2011), p. 139.
22	Roger Schultz, "Covenanting in America: The Political Theology of John Witherspoon," Master's Thesis, Trinity Evangelical Divinity School, Deerfield, Illinois, 1985, pp. 136-137. Quoted in Jerry Newcombe, D. Min., *Answers from the Founding Fathers*, (Fort Lauderdale, FL: Truth in Action Ministries, 2011), p. 135.
23	The Federalist No. 47, "The Particular Structure of the New Government and the Distribution of Power Among Its Different Parts." http://www.constitution.org/fed/federa47.htm.
24	Peter Orszag, "Too Much of a Good Thing: Why we need less democracy," *The New Republic*, September 14, 2011. http://www.tnr.com/article/politics/magazine/94940/peter-orszag-democracy.
25	Emily P. Walker, "AHIP: Politicos Talk Health Reform to Insurers," *Medpage

Today, June 16, 2011. http://www.medpagetoday.com/Washington-Watch/Reform/27110.
26 Jeffrey H. Anderson, "IPAB: Obama's Solution to Our 'Unfortunately' Democratic System," WeeklyStandard.com, June 17, 2011. http://www.weeklystandard.com/blogs/ipab-obama-s-solution-our-unfortunately-democratic-system_574797.html.
27 Avik Roy, "Donald Berwick Bows Out," NationalReview.com, Nov. 29, 2011. http://www.nationalreview.com/articles/284204/donald-berwick-bows-out-avik-roy.
28 George Will, "Government by the 'experts,'" June 10, 2011, *Washington Post*. http://www.washingtonpost.com/opinions/government-by-the-experts/2011/06/09/AGpU1KPH_story.html.
29 Paul Starr, *The Social Transformation of American Medicine: The Rise of a Sovereign Profession and the Making of a Vast Industry* (New York: Basic Books, 1982), p. 235. Quoted in Turner, Grace-Marie; Capretta, James C.; Miller, Thomas P.; Moffit, Robert E. *Why Obamacare Is Wrong for America: How the New Health Care Law Drives Up Costs, Puts Government in Charge of Your Decisions, and Threatens Your Constitutional Rights*. (City: Harper Collins, Inc., Kindle edition, 2011), p. 24.
30 Richard M. Ebeling, "Marching to Bismarck's Drummer: The Origins of the Modern Welfare State," *The Freeman: Ideas on Liberty*, December 2007. http://www.thefreemanonline.org/columns/from-the-president/marching-to-bismarcks-drummer-the-origins-of-the-modern-welfare-state/.
31 Grace-Marie Turner; James C. Capretta; Thomas P. Miller; Robert E. Moffit, *Why Obamacare Is Wrong for America: How the New Health Care Law Drives Up Costs, Puts Government in Charge of Your Decisions, and Threatens Your Constitutional Rights*, (City: Harper Collins, Inc., Kindle edition, 2011), p. 60.
32 "About the NHS," http://www.nhs.uk/NHSEngland/thenhs/about/Pages/overview.aspx.
33 Truth in Action Ministries interview with Wesley J. Smith, Nov. 21, 2011.
34 Jenny Hope and Nick Mcdermott, "The babies born in hospital corridors: Bed shortage forces 4,000 mothers to give birth in lifts, offices and hospital toilets," *Daily Mail*, August 26, 2009. http://www.dailymail.co.uk/news/article-1209034/The-babies-born-hospital-corridors-Bed-shortage-forces-4-000-mothers-birth-lifts-offices-hospital-toilets.html.
35 Oliver Wright, "Cataracts, hips, knees and tonsils: NHS begins rationing operations," *The Independent*, July 28, 2011. http://www.independent.co.uk/life-style/health-and-families/health-news/cataracts-hips-knees-and-tonsils-nhs-begins-rationing-operations-2327268.html.
36 Sarah Boseley, "Patients pull own teeth as dental contract falters," *The Guardian*, October 14, 2007. http://www.guardian.co.uk/uk/2007/oct/15/health.healthandwellbeing. Cited in Amy Ridenour and Ryan Balis, *Shattered Lives: 100 Victims of Government Health Care*, (Washington, D.C.: National Center for Public Policy Research, 2009), p. 35ff.
37 Martin Beckford, "NHS 'creaking at the seams' as waiting lists rise," *The Telegraph*, July 15, 2011. http://www.telegraph.co.uk/health/healthnews/8637738/NHS-creaking-at-the-seams-as-waiting-lists-rise.html.
38 Nick Ottens, "Health Care Waiting Lists in Britain Growing Longer," Atlantic Sentinel.com, May 23, 2011. http://atlanticsentinel.com/2011/05/health-care-waiting-lists-in-britain-growing-longer/.
39 Sally C. Pipes, *The Truth About Obamacare* (Washington, D.C., Regnery

Publishing, 2010), p. 127.
40 Martin Beckford, "Leukaemia sufferers denied drugs available in Scotland," *The Telegraph*, May 6, 2011. http://www.telegraph.co.uk/health/healthnews/8495374/Leukaemia-sufferers-denied-drugs-available-in-Scotland.html. Cited in Wesley Smith, "NHS Meltdown: NICE Rations Lifesaving Leukemia Drug," *Secondhand Smoke*, May 5, 2011. http://www.firstthings.com/blogs/secondhandsmoke/2011/05/05/nhs-meltdown-nice-rations-lifesaving-leukemia-drug/.
41 "… Nonetheless, with unrivaled ties to both Capitol Hill and the White House, he [Daschle] has remained an influential player in the debate over a health care overhaul. Mr. Daschle speaks frequently to President Obama, and many of the president's top advisers were once on Mr. Daschle's staff." Note last updated Aug. 24, 2009 on *New York Times* website at http://topics.nytimes.com/top/reference/timestopics/people/d/tom_daschle/index.html.
42 Dr. Scott Gottlieb, "Congress Wants to Restrict Drug Access," *Wall Street Journal*, January 20, 2009. http://online.wsj.com/article/SB123241385775896265.html?mod=googlenews_wsj.
43 Sandro Contenta, "Canadian health care has a dirty secret," *Global Post*, March 3, 2010. http://www.globalpost.com/dispatch/canada/100302/health-care-danny-williams.
44 Bacchus Barua, Mark Rovere, and Brett J. Skinner, *Waiting Your Turn: Wait Times for Health Care in Canada, 2010 Report*, Fraser Institute, p. 6.
45 "Dying on a Wait List?," August 6, 2009. http://factcheck.org/2009/08/dying-on-a-wait-list/.
46 "Health Care 'Reform' Puts Lives At Risk," *Impact*, August 2009. Newsletter of Truth in Action Ministries, formerly Coral Ridge Ministries.
47 Sally C. Pipes, *The Truth About Obamacare* (Washington, D.C., Regnery Publishing, 2010), p. 12. Also see "OECD Health Data 2011—Frequently Requested Data"; Excel file available to download at: http://www.oecd.org/document/16/0,3343,en_2649_34631_2085200_1_1_1_1,00.html.
48 Brett J. Skinner, "Hidden costs of Canadian health care system," Fraser Institute, July 17, 2007. http://www.fraserinstitute.org/publicationdisplay.aspx?id=11640&terms=doctor+shortage.
49 Peter Ferrara, *The Obamacare Disaster: An Appraisal of the Patient Protection and Affordable Care Act* (Chicago: The Heartland Institute, 2010) p. 44.
50 Ibid.
51 "Oregon Offers Terminal Patients Doctor-Assisted Suicide Instead of Medical Care," Foxnews.com, July 28, 2008. http://www.foxnews.com/story/0,2933,392962,00.html#ixzz1fU8n5qn1.
52 "State denies cancer treatment, offers suicide instead," WorldNetDaily.com, June 9, 2008. http://www.wnd.com/?pageId=67565.
53 Ibid.
54 Angelo S. Lynn, "Editorial: Political pragmatism is key to Vt.'s health care reform," *Addison County Independent*, July 18, 2011. http://www.addisonindependent.com/201107editorial-political-pragmatism-key-vts-health-care-reform.
55 Truth in Action Ministries interview with Wesley J. Smith, Nov. 21, 2011.
56 Liz Kowalczyk, "Across Mass., wait to see doctors grows," *Boston Globe*, September 22, 2008. http://www.boston.com/news/health/articles/2008/09/22/across_mass_wait_to_see_doctors_grows/.
57 Doug Bandow, "Romney Health Plan a Bust for Massachusetts,"

	RealClearPolitics.com, September 22, 2011. http://www.realclearpolitics.com/articles/2011/09/22/romney_health_plan_a_bust_for_massachusetts_111436.html.
58	Ibid.
59	Grace-Marie Turner and Amy Menefee, "Does Massachusetts Have a Miracle Cure for Health Reform?" Galen Institute, March 23, 2009. http://www.galen.org/component,8/action,show_content/id,13/blog_id,1178/category_id,8/type,33/. Cited in Peter Ferrara, *The Obamacare Disaster: An Appraisal of the Patient Protection and Affordable Care Act*, (Chicago: The Heartland Institute, 2010), p. 21.
60	Kay Lazar, "Costly ER Still Draws Many Now Insured," *Boston Globe*, April 24, 2009; Quoted in Peter Ferrara, *The Obamacare Disaster: An Appraisal of the Patient Protection and Affordable Care Act*, (Chicago: The Heartland Institute, 2010), p. 21.
61	Sally C. Pipes, *The Truth About Obamacare* (Washington, D.C.: Regnery Publishing, 2010), p. 96.
62	Timothy P. Cahill, "Massachusetts Is Our Future," *Wall Street Journal*, March 25, 2010. http://online.wsj.com/article/SB10001424052748704094104575144372942933394.html. Cited in Sally C. Pipes, *The Truth About Obamacare* (Washington, D.C.: Regnery Publishing, 2010), p. 97.
63	Doug Bandow, "Romney Health Plan a Bust for Massachusetts," RealClearPolitics.com, September 22, 2011. http://www.realclearpolitics.com/articles/2011/09/22/romney_health_plan_a_bust_for_massachusetts_111436.html.
64	"Rethinking Comparative Effectiveness Research," *Biotechnology Healthcare*, June 2009. http://www.ncbi.nlm.nih.gov/pmc/articles/PMC2799075/.
65	Henry Aaron and William B. Schwartz, "Rationing Health Care: The Choice Before Us," reprinted in *Emerging Issues in Biomedical Policy: An Annual Review*. Robert H. Blank, Andrea L. Bonnicksen, editors (New York: Columbia University Press, 1992), p. 58. Reprinted from Henry Aaron and William B. Schwartz, "Rationing Health Care: The Choice Before Us," *Science* 247:418-422, January 26, 1990. Cited in M. Catharine Evans, "For New Obama Nominee, Rationing Health Care Takes On Whole New Meaning," AmericanThinker.com, Nov. 19, 2011. http://www.americanthinker.com/blog/2011/11/for_new_obama_nominee_rationing_health_care_takes_on_whole_new_meaning.html#ixzz1fVuJk3bZ.
66	M. Catharine Evans, "For New Obama Nominee, Rationing Health Care Takes On Whole New Meaning," AmericanThinker.com, Nov. 19, 2011. http://www.americanthinker.com/blog/2011/11/for_new_obama_nominee_rationing_health_care_takes_on_whole_new_meaning.html#ixzz1fVuJk3bZ.
67	Henry Aaron, "IPAB repeal not warranted," Politico.com, July 14, 2011. http://www.politico.com/news/stories/0711/58993.html.
68	Tom Fitton, "Judicial Watch Obtains Documents Detailing ObamaCare Rationing," BigGovernment.com, April 6, 2011. http://biggovernment.com/tfitton/2011/04/06/judicial-watch-obtains-documents-detailing-obamacare-rationing/.
69	"The Avastin Mugging," *The Wall Street Journal*, August 18, 2010, http://online.wsj.com/article/SB10001424052748704271804575405203894857436.html.
70	Sally C. Pipes, *The Truth About Obamacare* (Washington, D.C.: Regnery Publishing, 2010), p. 129.
71	Peter Ferrara, *The Obamacare Disaster: An Appraisal of the Patient Protection*

72   *and Affordable Care Act*, (Chicago: The Heartland Institute, 2010), p. 18.
Gardiner Harris, "U.S. Panel Says No to Prostate Screening for Healthy Men," *New York Times*, October 6, 2011. http://www.nytimes.com/2011/10/07/health/07prostate.html?scp=1&sq=P.S.A.%20test%20task%20force&st=cse.
73   Press release, "Country's Largest Urology Group Defends the Need for Prostate Cancer Screening and Early Detection," Marketwatch.com, Oct. 7, 2011. http://www.marketwatch.com/story/countrys-largest-urology-group-defends-the-need-for-prostate-cancer-screening-and-early-detection-2011-10-07.
74   Spencer Harris, "The Rationing Begins," Texas Public Policy Foundation, October 11, 2011. http://www.texaspolicy.com/legislativeupdates_single.php?report_id=4120.
75   Shari Rudavsky, "Should men get the PSA test?" *Indianapolis Star*, Nov. 19, 2011. http://www.indystar.com/article/20111120/LIVING01/111200314/Should-men-get-PSA-test-?odyssey=tab%7Ctopnews%7Ctext%7CLiving.
76   Peter Ferrara, *The Obamacare Disaster: An Appraisal of the Patient Protection and Affordable Care Act*, (Chicago: The Heartland Institute, 2010), p. 12.
77   "2011 Annual Report of the Boards of Trustees of the Federal Hospital Insurance and Federal Supplementary Medical Insurance Trust Funds," p. 4. https://www.cms.gov/ReportsTrustFunds/downloads/tr2011.pdf.
78   Statement by Richard S. Foster, Chief Actuary, Centers for Medicare & Medicaid Services, U.S. Department of Health and Human Services (HHS) on The Estimated Effect of the Affordable Care Act on Medicare and Medicaid Outlays and Total National Health Care Expenditures, May 16, 2011. http://www.hhs.gov/asl/testify/2011/03/t20110330e.html.
79   Senate Budget Committee, Minority Staff, "Budget Perspective: The Real Deficit Effect of the Democrats' Health Package," March 23, 2010. Cited in Peter Ferrara, *The Obamacare Disaster: An Appraisal of the Patient Protection and Affordable Care Act*, (Chicago: The Heartland Institute, 2010), p. 12.
80   Grace-Marie Turner, "Testimony before the U.S. House of Representatives Committee on the Budget, Hearing on Medicare's Future: An Examination of the Independent Payment Advisory Board," July 12, 2011.
81   Peter Ferrara, *The Obamacare Disaster: An Appraisal of the Patient Protection and Affordable Care Act*, (Chicago: The Heartland Institute, 2010), p. 12.
82   Richard S. Foster, Chief Actuary, "Estimated Financial Effects of the 'Patient Protection and Affordable Care Act,' as Amended," Centers for Medicare and Medicaid Services, April 22, 2010, p. 10. https://www.cms.gov/ActuarialStudies/downloads/PPACA_2010-04-22.pdf.
83   Peter Ferrara, *The Obamacare Disaster: An Appraisal of the Patient Protection and Affordable Care Act*, (Chicago: The Heartland Institute, 2010), p. 12.
84   David Olmos, "Mayo Clinic in Arizona to Stop Treating Some Medicare Patients," Bloomberg, Dec. 31, 2009. http://www.bloomberg.com/apps/news?pid=newsarchive&sid=aHoYSI84VdL0.
85   Peter Ferrara, *The Obamacare Disaster: An Appraisal of the Patient Protection and Affordable Care Act*, (Chicago: The Heartland Institute, 2010), p. 14.
86   Ibid., pp. 13-14.
87   Ibid., p. 16.
88   Jeffrey H. Anderson, "Obamacare Ends Construction of Doctor-Owned Hospitals," Weeklystandard.com, Jan. 3, 2011. http://www.weeklystandard.com/blogs/obamacare-ends-construction-doctor-owned-hospitals_525950.html.
89   Kenneth Artz, "Physician-Owned Hospitals Fire Back at Obamacare

Restrictions," Heartland Institute. http://news.heartland.org/newspaper-article/physician-owned-hospitals-fire-back-obamacare-restrictions.

90 "Physician Hospitals of America Survey: Affordable Care Act Blocks 6300 Jobs & $1.8 Billion in Construction Spending," Nov. 29, 2011 press release. http://www.marketwatch.com/story/physician-hospitals-of-america-survey-affordable-care-act-blocks-6300-jobs-18-billion-in-construction-spending-2011-11-29.

91 Peter Ferrara, *The Obamacare Disaster: An Appraisal of the Patient Protection and Affordable Care Act*, (Chicago: The Heartland Institute, 2010), p. 16.

92 "Text of Obama Speech on the Deficit," *The Wall Street Journal*, April 13, 2011. http://blogs.wsj.com/washwire/2011/04/13/text-of-obama-speech-on-the-deficit/.

93 Michelle Malkin, "Rolling Back the Obamacare Banana Republic," NationalReview.com, July 13, 2011. http://www.nationalreview.com/articles/271744/rolling-back-obamacare-banana-republic-michelle-malkin.

94 Jennifer Haberkorn, "Medicare pay board is losing vital support," Politico.com, June 8, 2011. http://www.politico.com/news/stories/0611/56467.html.

95 Janice Shaw Crouse, "IPAB: The Independent Payment Advisory Board—Rationing the Life Out of You," *Family Voice Insight*, August 2011 (publication of Concerned Women for America), p. 5.

96 Stanley Kurtz, "IPAB, Obama, and Socialism," NationalReview.com, April 18, 2011. http://www.nationalreview.com/corner/264988/ipab-obama-and-socialism-stanley-kurtz.

97 Michelle Malkin, "Rolling Back the Obamacare Banana Republic," NationalReview.com, July 13, 2011. http://www.nationalreview.com/articles/271744/rolling-back-obamacare-banana-republic-michelle-malkin.

98 "CRS Confirms White House Could Recess Appoint Controversial Medicare Czars," website of Sen. Tom Coburn, March 21, 2011. http://coburn.senate.gov/public/index.cfm/rightnow?ContentRecord_id=3238f6b5-cb13-409f-81e0-f143525a0ed5&ContentType_id=b4672ca4-3752-49c3-bffc-fd099b51c966&Group_id=00380921-999d-40f6-a8e3-470468762340&MonthDisplay=3&YearDisplay=2011.

99 Public law 111-148, "Patient Protection and Affordable Care Act," Sec. 3403.

100 Jack Ebeler, Tricia Neuman and Juliette Cubanski, "The Independent Payment Advisory Board: A New Approach To Controlling Medicare Spending," The Henry J. Kaiser Family Foundation, April 2011, p. 6.

101 As of Dec. 10, 2011. See http://thomas.loc.gov/home/thomas.php.

102 Sam Baker, "270 healthcare groups back IPAB repeal," TheHill.com, June 24, 2011. http://thehill.com/blogs/healthwatch/health-reform-implementation/168407-270-healthcare-groups-back-ipab-repeal.

103 Andrew Stiles, "Is IPAB Repeal in the Cards?" NationalReview.com, June 13, 2011. http://www.nationalreview.com/articles/269429/ipab-repeal-cards-andrew-stiles?pg=1.

104 Ibid.

105 Truth in Action Ministries interview with Wesley J. Smith, Nov. 21, 2011.

106 Michelle Malkin, "Rolling Back the Obamacare Banana Republic," *National Review*, July 13, 2011. http://www.nationalreview.com/articles/271744/rolling-back-obamacare-banana-republic-michelle-malkin.

107 "IPAB: The Controversial Consequences for Medicare and Seniors," Testimony of Diane Cohen, Senior Attorney, Goldwater Institute, Phoenix, Arizona, Before the United States House of Representatives Committee on Energy

	and Commerce Subcommittee of Health, July 14, 2011. http://republicans.energycommerce.house.gov/Media/file/Hearings/Health/071311/Cohen.pdf.
108	Mark Hemingway, "The Real Mediscare: Obama's rationing is the thing to worry about," *The Weekly Standard*, May 9, 2011. http://www.weeklystandard.com/articles/real-mediscare_558502.html?page=1.
109	42 USCS § 1395kkk(g)(1)(B)(i)
110	Sally C. Pipes, *The Truth About Obamacare* (Washington, D.C.: Regnery Publishing, 2010), pp. 149-150.
111	Jack Ebeler, Tricia Neuman and Juliette Cubanski, "The Independent Payment Advisory Board: A New Approach To Controlling Medicare Spending," The Henry J. Kaiser Family Foundation, April 2011, p. 10.
112	Ibid.
113	James Gutman, "IPAB Stirs Major New Fears in MA Industry; Board's Impact Could Hit Smaller Plans Hard," *Medicare Advantage News*, June 30, 2011. http://aishealth.com/archive/nman063011-01.
114	Sally C. Pipes, *The Truth About Obamacare* (Washington, D.C.: Regnery Publishing, 2010), pp. 48, 147.
115	Michael Warren, "Sebelius Doubles Down on IPAB Defense," *The Weekly Standard*, July 13, 2011. http://www.weeklystandard.com/blogs/sebelius-doubles-down-ipab-defense_576812.html.
116	Peter Ferrara, *The Obamacare Disaster: An Appraisal of the Patient Protection and Affordable Care Act,* (Chicago: The Heartland Institute, 2010), Location 49 on Kindle edition.
117	Henry J. Aaron, "The Independent Payment Advisory Board — Congress's 'Good Deed,'" *The New England Journal of Medicine*, June 23, 2011. http://www.nejm.org/doi/full/10.1056/NEJMp1105144.
118	"Text of Obama Speech on the Deficit," *The Wall Street Journal*, April 13, 2011. http://blogs.wsj.com/washwire/2011/04/13/text-of-obama-speech-on-the-deficit/.
119	Ibid.
120	Grace-Marie Turner, President, Galen Institute, "An Examination of the Independent Payment Advisory Board," Testimony before the U.S. House of Representatives Committee on the Budget, Rep. Paul Ryan, Chairman, Hearing on Medicare's Future, July 12, 2011, p. 7. http://budget.house.gov/UploadedFiles/Turner_Testimony.pdf.
121	"FACT SHEET: The President's Framework for Shared Prosperity and Shared Fiscal Responsibility," The White House, April 13, 2011. http://www.whitehouse.gov/the-press-office/2011/04/13/fact-sheet-presidents-framework-shared-prosperity-and-shared-fiscal-resp.
122	Grace-Marie Turner, President, Galen Institute, "An Examination of the Independent Payment Advisory Board," Testimony before the U.S. House of Representatives Committee on the Budget, Rep. Paul Ryan, Chairman, Hearing on Medicare's Future, July 12, 2011, p. 7.
123	Jackie Calmes, "After Health Care Passage, Obama Pushes to Get It Rolling," *New York Times*, April 17, 2010. http://www.nytimes.com/2010/04/18/health/policy/18cost.html.
124	Allen Dobson, Joan DaVanzo and Namrata Sen, "The Cost-Shift Payment 'Hydraulic': Foundation, History, and Implications," *Health Affairs*, 25, no. 1 (2006): 22-33. http://content.healthaffairs.org/content/25/1/22.full. Cited in Sally C. Pipes, *The Truth About Obamacare* (Washington, D.C., Regnery Publishing, 2010), p. 80.

125	Timothy Stoltzfus Jost, J.D., "The Independent Payment Advisory Board," *The New England Journal of Medicine*, 363:103-105, July 8, 2010. http://www.nejm.org/doi/full/10.1056/NEJMp1005402.
126	Public law 111-148, "Patient Protection and Affordable Care Act," Sec. 3403.
127	Jack Ebeler, Tricia Neuman and Juliette Cubanski, "The Independent Payment Advisory Board: A New Approach To Controlling Medicare Spending," The Henry J. Kaiser Family Foundation, April 2011, p. 9.
128	"How The Obama Health Law Will Ration Your Family's Medical Treatment," Robert Powell Center for Medical Ethics at the National Right to Life Committee. See http://www.nrlc.org/healthcarerationing/ObamaHCRationingBasicDOCUMENTATION.pdf.
129	NRLC note states:

Understanding the legislative language that sets the required target below the rate of medical inflation requires following a very convoluted path: 42 USCS § 1395kkk(o) states,

"Advisory recommendations for non-Federal health care programs. (1) In general. Not later than January 15, 2015, and at least once every two years thereafter, the Board shall submit to Congress and the President recommendations to slow the growth in national health expenditures (excluding expenditures under this title and in other Federal health care programs) ... such as recommendations-- (A) that the Secretary or other Federal agencies can implement administratively; ... (2) Coordination. In making recommendations under paragraph (1), the Board shall coordinate such recommendations with recommendations contained in proposals and advisory reports produced by the Board under subsection (c)."

The reference is to 42 USCS § 1395kkk(c)(2)(A)(i), which provides for Board reports with recommendations that "will result in a net reduction in total Medicare program spending in the implementation year that is at least equal to the applicable savings target established under paragraph (7)(B) for such implementation year."

The "applicable savings target" is whatever is the lesser of two alternative targets [42 USCS § 1395kkk(c)(7)(B)].

First alternative: 2015 through 2017: The reduction necessary to limit the growth in medical spending to equal a percentage halfway between medical inflation and general inflation (using 5-year averages) [42 USCS § 1395kkk(c)(6)(C)(I)].

In 2018 and later years: The reduction necessary to limit the growth in medical spending to "the nominal gross domestic product per capita plus 1.0 percentage point" [42USCS § 1395kkk(c)(6)(C)(ii)].

Second alternative: The reduction necessary to force actual spending below projected spending by a specified percentage of projected medical spending; the specified percentage differs by year (in 2015, .5%; in 2016, 1%; in 2017, 1.25%; in 2018 and in subsequent years, 1.5%)[42 USCS § 1395kkk(c)(7)(C)(I)].

130	NRLC note states:

This provision is quoted at the beginning of endnote [129] above.

131	NRLC note states:

42 USCS § 1395l (t)(17) ["Each subsection (d) hospital shall submit data on measures selected under this paragraph to the Secretary in a form and manner, and at a time, specified by the Secretary for purposes of this paragraph"....and "(A) Reduction in update for failure to report. (i) In general

... a subsection (d) hospital ... that does not submit, to the Secretary in accordance with this paragraph, data required to be submitted on measures selected under this paragraph with respect to such a year, the ... fee schedule increase factor ... for such year shall be reduced by 2.0 percentage points."], 1395l(i)(7) [similar language applicable to ambulatory surgical centers], 1395cc(k)(3) [similar language applicable to certain cancer hospitals], 1395rr(h)(2)(A)(iii) [similar language applicable to end-stage renal disease programs], 1395ww(b)(3)(B)(viii) [similar language otherwise applicable to hospitals], (j)(7)(D) [similar language applicable to inpatient rehabilitation hospitals], (m)(5)(D) [similar language applicable to long-term care hospitals], (s)(4)(D) [similar language applicable to psychiatric hospitals], and 1395fff(b)(3)(B)(v) [similar language applicable to skilled nursing facilities], 1395(i)(5)(D) [similar language applicable to hospice care], and (o)(2) [applicable to the way in which value-based incentives are paid].

132 NRLC note states:
    42 USCS § 18031(h)(1) provides, "Beginning on January 1, 2015, a qualified health plan may contract with ... (B) a health care provider only if such provider implements such mechanisms to improve health care quality as the Secretary may by regulation require."

133 Wesley J. Smith, "Obamacare: Robert Reich Tells "the Truth" About the Downsides of Health Care Reform," *Secondhand Smoke*, Oct. 13, 2009. http://www.firstthings.com/blogs/secondhandsmoke/2009/10/13/obamacare-robert-reich-tells-the-truth-about-the-downsides-of-health-care-reform/.

134 Sarah Palin, "Statement on the Current Health Care Debate," Facebook, Aug. 7, 2009. http://www.facebook.com/note.php?note_id=113851103434.

135 Brett Coughlin, "Politics trump policy on 'death panels,'" Politico.com, January 5, 2011. http://www.politico.com/news/stories/0111/47117.html.

136 Jim Rutenberg and Jackie Calmes, "False 'Death Panel' Rumor Has Some Familiar Roots," *New York Times*, August 13, 2009. http://www.nytimes.com/2009/08/14/health/policy/14panel.html.

137 Jon Meacham, "I Was a Teenage Death Panelist," *Newsweek*, September 11, 2009. http://www.thedailybeast.com/newsweek/2009/09/11/i-was-a-teenage-death-panelist.html.

138 Evan Thomas, "The Case for Killing Granny," *Newsweek*, September 11, 2009. http://www.thedailybeast.com/newsweek/2009/09/11/the-case-for-killing-granny.html.

139 "Is Newer Better? Not Always," *The New York Times*, September 11, 2010. http://www.nytimes.com/2010/09/12/opinion/12sun1.html?_r=1&ref=opinion.

140 Richard D. Lamm, "Lamm: Rationing could fix health care," *Denver Post*, June 26, 2011. http://www.denverpost.com/opinion/ci_18341751#ixzz1fxhnDahZ.

141 Jane E. Allen, "Two Dead Since Arizona Medicaid Program Slashed Transplant Coverage," ABC News, January 6, 2011. http://abcnews.go.com/Health/News/arizona-transplant-deaths/story?id=12559369.

142 Wesley J. Smith, "About Those Death Panels ...," *The Weekly Standard*, January 31, 2011. http://www.weeklystandard.com/articles/about-those-death-panels_536874.html?page=1.

143 Truth in Action Ministries interview with Wesley J. Smith, Nov. 21, 2011.

144 Charles Colson and Nancy Pearcey, *How Now Shall We Live?* (Wheaton, IL: Tyndale House Publishers, Inc., 1999), p. 118.

145 Wesley J. Smith, "Death by Ethics Committee," *National Review*, April 27, 2006.

	http://old.nationalreview.com/smithw/smith200604271406.asp.
146	John Hardwig, "Is There A Duty To Die?" *Hastings Center Report*, 27, no. 2 (1997): 34-42. http://web.utk.edu/~jhardwig/dutydie.htm.
147	Ibid.
148	Martin Beckford, "Baroness Warnock: Dementia sufferers may have a 'duty to die,'" *The Telegraph*, Sept. 18, 2008. http://www.telegraph.co.uk/news/uknews/2983652/Baroness-Warnock-Dementia-sufferers-may-have-a-duty-to-die.html.
149	Ibid.
150	Alvin J. Schmidt, *How Christianity Changed the World* (Grand Rapids, MI: Zondervan, 2001, 2004), p. 128.
151	Ibid., p. 129.
152	Ibid., p. 153.
153	D. James Kennedy and Jerry Newcombe, *What If Jesus Had Never Been Born?* (Nashville, TN: Thomas Nelson Publishers, Inc., 1994), p. 9.
154	Alvin J. Schmidt, *How Christianity Changed the World* (Grand Rapids, MI: Zondervan, 2001, 2004), p. 155.
155	Ibid., p. 167.
156	Ibid., p. 152.
157	Ibid.
158	Ibid., p. 155.
159	Ibid., p. 156. Also see D. James Kennedy and Jerry Newcombe, *What If Jesus Had Never Been Born?* (Nashville, TN: Thomas Nelson Publishers, Inc., 1994), p. 146.
160	Schmidt, p. 157.
161	Ibid.
162	Kennedy and Newcombe, p. 149.
163	Ibid., p. 151.
164	Ibid., p. 152.
165	Truth in Action Ministries interview with Wesley J. Smith, Nov. 21, 2011.
166	Grace-Marie Turner; James C. Capretta; Thomas P. Miller; Robert E. Moffit, *Why Obamacare Is Wrong for America: How the New Health Care Law Drives Up Costs, Puts Government in Charge of Your Decisions, and Threatens Your Constitutional Rights* (City: Harper Collins, 2011, Kindle edition), p. 59.
167	C.S. Lewis, *God in the Dock, Essays on Theology and Ethics*. Edited by Walter Hooper. (Grand Rapids, MI: Eerdmans, 1970), p. 199. Quoted in *The Quotable Lewis*, Wayne Martindale, Jerry Lewis, Editors (Wheaton, Illinois: Tyndale House, 1990), p. 479.